A B C OF ADLER'S PSYCHOLOGY

Founded by C. K. Ogden

The International Library of Psychology

INDIVIDUAL DIFFERENCES
In 21 Volumes

A B C OF ADLER'S PSYCHOLOGY

PHILIPPE MAIRET

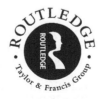

First published in 1928 by
Kegan Paul, Trench, Trubner & Co., Ltd.

Reprinted 1999, 2000, 2001 by
Routledge

2 Park Square, Milton Park, Abingdon, Oxfordshire OX14 4RN
711 Third Avenue, New York, NY 10017

Transferred to Digital Printing 2006

Routledge is an imprint of the Taylor and Francis Group, an informa company

© 1928 Philippe Mairet

British Library Cataloguing in Publication Data
A CIP catalogue record for this book
is available from the British Library

A B C of Adler's Psychology
ISBN 13: 978-0-415-21064-5 (hbk)
ISBN 13: 978-0-415-75812-3 (pbk)

Individual Differences: 21 Volumes
ISBN 978-0-415-21130-7
The International Library of Psychology: 204 Volumes
ISBN 978-0-415-19132-6

CONTENTS

FOREWORD

Individual Psychology is not psycho-analysis. It is a method, initiated by Dr Adler of Vienna, of gaining knowledge of individuals, including knowledge of their inner life, but it is a method founded upon a view of the individual as whole in himself, an indivisible unit of human society. It relates everything that the individual does in such a way as to obtain a picture of a single, coherent and intelligible tendency, expressed in most various ways, direct and indirect. Thus it is a method of unifying the psyche much more than of dissecting it. Even the distinction between ' conscious ' and ' unconscious ' mind is not fully admitted by Adler. " The unconscious is much less unconscious than we suppose," he says, " and the conscious much less conscious."

Thus, while it has grown up as part of that revolution in modern psychology which is called psycho-analysis, Individual Psychology is definitely opposed to analysis merely as such, and only uses analysis in the service of synthesis. It has been advisable, in this brief survey, to touch upon certain points of controversy, not at all to repudiate Adler's relation with the whole development of psycho-analytic knowledge, but to define the unique and characteristic aim with which he uses it.

This book attempts only to give the leading ideas of Individual Psychology, and a sketch of their origins. It is meant for the general reader who may be aware that he, like everyone else, is a psychologist in practice, however unsystematic. Even the few proven principles here outlined would be, if applied to experience with sufficient alertness and elasticity of mind, of great help to the practical knowledge of human nature. In order to gain an adequate understanding of this subject, however, it is necessary to read Dr Adler's works, "Individual Psychology," and "The Neurotic Constitution," which are translated into English. There is also a large and growing literature of his colleagues in Germany and Austria, which shows the application of his principles in many other spheres of life as well as in the art of healing.

A B C OF
ADLER'S PSYCHOLOGY

CHAPTER I

THE BASIS OF MODERN PSYCHOLOGY

DR ALFRED ADLER'S work in psychology, while it is scientific and general in method, is essentially the study of the separate personalities we are, and is 'herefore called Individual Psychology. Concrete, particular, unique human beings are the subjects of this psychology, and it can only be truly learned from the men, women and children we meet.

The supreme importance of this contribution to modern psychology is due to the manner in which it reveals how all the activities of the soul are drawn together into the service of the individual, how all his faculties and strivings are related to one end. We are enabled by this to enter into the ideals, the difficulties, the efforts and discouragements of our fellow-men, in such a way that we may obtain a whole and living picture of each as a personality. In this co-ordinating idea, something like finality is achieved, though we must understand it as finality of foundation. There has never before been a method so rigorous and yet adaptable for following the fluctuations of that most fluid, variable and elusive of all realities, the individual human soul.

Since Adler regards not only science but even intelligence itself as the result of the communal efforts of humanity, we shall find his consciousness of his own unique contribution more than usually tempered by recognition of his collaborators, both past and contemporary. It will therefore be useful to consider Adler's relation to the movement called Psycho-analysis, and first of all to recall, however briefly, the philosophic impulses which inspired the psycho-analytic movement as a whole.

It may be said without exaggeration that psycho-analysis owes its existence to Schopenhauer. The most important psycho-analysts admit a direct debt to him ; but their indirect income from him is much greater, for his forcible reversal of the tendency of European thought is responsible for various other movements which have converged upon modern psychology. Schopenhauer's importance in this respect is not due to his psychological observations, penetrating as they often are, but to his exaltation of the *Will* into the first principle of his system. In all his writings it is the will and not the intelligence which is studied as the *magnum mysterium*. This Will, which is the immanent, omnipotent creator of everything, is made by Schopenhauer to appear much more like the devil than like God, for it is a blind urge to self-existence, utterly relentless in nature. Even the intelligence which it produces in Man, the highest order of its creation, is only produced in order to further its own aims. But in this the Will, as it were, over-reaches itself, for intelligence produces self-consciousness, which finally detects the evil of its own will. This Will does not really desire the good of its own creatures, but only their continuation, and not even their continuation as individuals, but through procreation as species. The individual thinks all the time that he is pursuing his own pleasure, but that is exactly how the Will manages him. Pleasure is like the carrot which the Irishman, sitting in the cart, dangles before the donkey's nose on a stick to make it go, and removes to make it stop. That is how the Will drives man, against his own true interest. When man's intellect, however, rises to the height of general conceptions, it can perceive itself in relation to all things, and then it realizes that it is only an instrument. It is as if the donkey perceived the stick that holds the carrot, and realized that it would never reach it.

Such a homely illustration gives no idea of the greatness of Schopenhauer's theme, but may roughly indicate how he focussed attention upon the mystery of the will. He inevitably led men to search for the vital impulses behind thoughts rather than for the inter-relations between thoughts themselves. This conception of the Will as a universal Will to live spread much further than Schopenhauer's own writings.

It ascended to be the Will to Power of Nietzsche and descended to be the "Life-Force" of Bernard Shaw. But it was through Eduard Von Hartmann that it took its most vital line of evolution.

Hartmann took his stand upon the indivisibility of Will and Idea. No idea is possible without Will and no movement of the Will exists which is not at the same time an idea. To Hartmann, therefore, it was absurd to conceive of the creative urge in the universe as "blind" Will, or even as Will in the abstract. It is very far-seeing and is just as much intelligence as will. A being may not be able to express its will in any other way than by action, but that does not prove that its will is not also an idea. A bird building its nest for the first time cannot translate its purpose into anything else *except* concrete reality, cannot express its idea in words or fantasy— probably not even to itself. But can it therefore be said to have no purpose, no idea? Clearly there is an idea dynamically present, but in a state which we call 'unconscious' because it is not translatable into words or symbols. The real Being of the Universe, realizing itself in all creation, including man and civilization, is precisely this unconscious force of intelligence. Not that it is correctly described as unconscious (Hartmann was inclined later to re-name his arch-concept " the Superconscious "), but to our limited consciousnesses, revolving in their own memory-films of words and images, this deeper substratum seems dark and inexpressible. The Unconscious is a much vaster, super-individual intelligence from which our conscious thinking has cut itself off.

This idea was to become the foundation of modern psychology. It suggested that the most important discoveries of the working of the mind were to be made at the deeper levels of consciousness—in fact, in the less clearly conscious states. In France especially, while Hartmann was being read with great appreciation, psychologists such as Janet and Charcot were experimenting with hypnotism. They found that a hypnotized subject, in a state resembling sleep, and unaware of his surroundings, could recall memories of which he was quite unconscious when normally awake. They also found that suggestions accepted in this condition were capable of influencing behaviour afterwards, although the patient had no conscious memory of accepting them.

These precise discoveries of the existence of unconscious memories and their activity in the life were of vast importance to psychology, and they are now placed beyond all question by ever-accumulating masses of evidence.

What we now call the " Unconscious " or the " Unconscious Mind " is conceived to be a vast and complicated structure of memory, of which only a working minimum is accessible to conscious recall. Much the greater part of memory continues to play its part in the individual's life in a transmuted form, not as recollection, but as feeling— as emotional reaction to things and persons. In that way it continually exercises more or less suggestive power, but it is difficult, and perhaps sometimes impossible, to recall it to consciousness in the form of the original impressions. It is easy to see that the earliest impressions must have naturally the most purely emotional strength, and this is, in fact, what all psycho-analysts find. The book of memory is not like a book with successive leaves, so much as a single tablet all over which the first impressions are scrawled in a large and simple style and the succeeding ones have to be written around them, till it is over-written again and again in smaller and smaller characters. This metaphor is only meant to suggest that all subsequent impressions have to be fitted into former ones. The actual process is fundamentally simple; whatever happens to an individual, he reacts to it according to his previous experience of the most successful way of meeting that kind of situation. He does not remember most of the memories that guide him, but they exert their united pressure by the emotional *tone* of aversion or inclination to certain actions. Should he encounter an entirely new situation, he will either have no idea how to deal with it, or he will relate it to the most similar experience he knows, probably to one of his earliest experiences which is not even much like it.

In this transformation of memory into emotion, we are confronted by a biological necessity; the greater part of memory must be changed into feeling in order to be serviceable to life. Emotion acts almost instantaneously, and with a tremendous range of discrimination, whereas the stock of recollections which we keep " indexed," as it were, serves a higher human purpose, but is both too cumbersome and too limited for immediate use. We cannot live by it, we cannot wait to read it up, and our emotional nature will not allow us to do so.

There are, unfortunately, such things as entirely mischievous emotional memories. These are memories which have been suppressed into the emotional form before their meaning to the individual has been at all understood. Such memories, thrust too soon out of consciousness, turn into emotional complexes which act in the reverse of a useful manner. The individual subject may then become a patient; he is either prevented from acting in what he sees to be a reasonable way, or else impelled to act unreasonably, by an emotional stress which he cannot himself understand, or which he explains to himself by a quite wrong " rationalization."

Such an unassimilable memory can be generally fished up again and brought into consciousness by the technique of psycho-analysis, in which case it ceases to be an emotional complex and becomes a more or less normal fact of the memory. The astonishing clearness with which forgotten memories can be restored by this means *whenever they are of vital importance* suggests that such memories never fade—they are only covered over. We owe this technique chiefly to Freud and his school, and much of the prestige of psycho-analysis was achieved by its apparently miraculous cures of war-neuroses, such as shell-shock.

Our modern view of the soul, then, reveals it as a vast reservoir of memories, which makes itself felt in every instant as the emotional reality of that instant. It is the living reality of the past, exerting a powerful influence upon the present through our feelings. Academic psychologists may still continue, half convinced, to derive the psyche from a dozen or so of " instincts " which are conceived almost as if they were metaphysical realities. But there is no need now for any metaphysical " instinct of self-assertion "—not even for a " sexual instinct." There are individuals who have proved what it is to *succeed* by submission, but there is no entity we can call the " submissive instinct " which uses individuals as its instruments. There are, however, individuals with a permanent policy of submissiveness, in whom it is possible to trace the emotional memories of success through their policy, and it can be found that they tend to seek out over and over again positions of dependence in which their proven policy will succeed.

This conception of the Unconscious as vital memory—biological memory—is common to modern psychology as a whole. But Freud, from the first a specialist in hysteria, took the memories of success or failure in the sexual life, as of the first— and almost the only—importance. Jung, a psychiatrist of genius, has tried to widen this distressingly narrow view, by seeking to reveal the super-individual or racial memories which, he believes, have as much power as the sexual and a higher kind of value for life.

It was left to Alfred Adler, a physician

of wide and general experience, to unite the conception of the Unconscious more firmly with biological reality. A man of the original school of psycho-analysts, he had done much work by that method of analyzing memories out of their coagulated emotional state into clearness and objectivity. But he showed that the whole scheme of memory is different in every individual. Individuals do not form their unconscious memories all around the same central motive—not all around sexuality, for instance. In every individual we find an individual way of selecting its experiences from all possible experience. What is the principle of that selectivity? Adler has answered that it is, fundamentally, the organic consciousness of a *need*, of some specific inferiority which has to be compensated. It is as though every soul had consciousness of its whole physical reality, and were concentrated, with sleepless insistence, upon achieving compensation for the defects in it.

Thus the whole life of the small man, for instance, would be interpretable as a struggle to achieve immediate greatness in some way, and that of a deaf man to obtain a compensation for not hearing. It is not so simple as that, of course, for a system of defects may give rise to a constellation of guiding ideas, and also in human life we have to deal with imaginary inferiorities and fantastic strivings, but even here the principle is the same.

The sexual life, far from controlling all activities, fits perfectly into the frame of those more important strivings, for it is pre-eminently under the control of emotion, and emotion is moulded by the entire vital history. Thus a Freudian analysis gives a true account of the sexual *consequences* of a given life-line, but it is a true *diagnosis* only in that sense.

Psychology becomes now for the first time rooted in biology. The tendencies of the soul, and the mind's development, are seen to be controlled from the first by the effort to compensate for organic defects or for positions of inferiority. Everything that is exceptional or individual in the disposition of an organic being originates in this way. The principle is common to man and animal, probably even to the vegetable kingdom also ; and the special endowments of species are to be taken as arising from experience of defects and inferiorities in relation to their environment, which has been successfully compensated by activity, growth and structure.

There is nothing new in the idea of compensation as a biological principle, for it has been long known that the body will over-develop certain parts in compensation for the injury of others. If one kidney ceases to function, for instance, the other develops abnormally until it does the work of both ; if the heart springs a leak in a valve; the whole organ grows larger to allow for its loss of efficiency, and when nervous tissue is destroyed, adjacent tissue of another kind endeavours to take on the nerve-function. The compensatory developments of the whole organism to meet the exigencies of any special work or exertion are too numerous and well known to need illustration. But it is Dr Adler who has first transferred this principle bodily to psychology as a fundamental idea, and demonstrated the part it plays in the soul and intellect.

Not that human psychology is a branch

of biology. The human organism is in a radically different situation from that of any other, in a position of much greater inferiority relative to Nature. Man is in the critical predicament of having to save his own being by the creation of the supra-biological organism, human society.

CHAPTER II

The Life Goal

Any one who quotes feelingly the verse. about " one far-off Divine event to which the whole Creation moves " is making what is called a " teleological " assumption about the universe. He is asserting that it has a *goal*. He means that all its present activity and being is a preparation for its final state, like a drama which was conceived and produced for the sake of its final scene. It is possible to take this teleological view of phenomena. They may just as well be conditioned by what they are going to be, as by what they have been.

But can we say that an individual being, a winged insect or a lion, for example, is moving towards *its own* " far-off Divine perfection "—towards a higher kind of its own existence? There is no usefulness in such an idea. It is certain that if the lion had a static vision or picture of a more glorious being which it was going to become, this would only be a hindrance to it. The way in which beings have attained their present perfection shows that no being is responsible for its own form, but all are mutually responsible. The entire form and functioning of a winged insect proceed from an evolution inextricably involved with that of plants it has lived upon and of birds and other insects that have preyed upon it. We are impressed by the apparent determination of every being to maintain its own *style of life*, but equally by its elasticity and adaptability to every change of circumstances. The teleological principle of individuals, if we can call it so, is something which is at the same time as fixed as possible and very adaptable. That is, it is a principle of compensation, sometimes even leading to over-compensation. We need not suppose that, in their original essence, any beings have an urge to life which is different from that of others, but in having had to compensate for different positions of inferiority they have become innumerably differentiated. Between all beings on the whole there is a living agreement, unity and reciprocity, which is maintained by their success in dealing with their own difficulties.

If an ass got the idea that he was going to become a unicorn, either himself by effort or his posterity by evolution, unicornness would not have become the true teleological principle of that ass. His behaviour, no doubt, would become peculiar, and might unfit him for life with his fellows, and might actually lead to death or degeneration. For, if our whole view of Nature is not mistaken, the ass could only really become a unicorn by the co-operation, friendly and hostile, of many other beings, ultimately of the whole of Nature, *as well as* by his own self-affirmation.

This is, of course, an unreal instance, since animals are not troubled by individual fantasies about their destiny. But in human life the individual fantasy plays a very important part for evil and for good. The Fall of Man is generally ascribed to his having had a fantasy of becoming a God. In a sense it may be said that Individual Psychology is the investigation of human fantasies. The first principle established by that science is that fantasy, which is invariably present, is always the compensation for a *feeling* of inferiority.

No psychic phenomenon, says Dr Adler, can be grasped and understood unless it is regarded as the preparation for some goal. The task of psychology is to understand all the movements and emotional phases of an individual, and to get the picture of an integrated life-plan and a final goal. This is as generally true for the mentally healthy subjects as for the diseased, and in neither case is the life-goal very consciously formulated. It is not, however, so much unconscious as *secret*. The greatest efforts will be made to preserve that secret, even in the face of the most benevolent enquiry, and in spite of great distress caused by the concealment of it. That is the reason for the immense difficulty of practical psychology and the subtlety of its technique. The secret has come to be of vital importance. Let us recall what was said in the preceding chapter about biological memories and their permanence in the emotional disposition. The secret life-goal of the individual must be conceived as having been

elaborated to compensate the chief inferiority : it has therefore all the strength
of life behind it—or rather in front of it,
to protect it, to defend it. When we say
to a man, in reproof of some particularly
outrageous piece of behaviour, " Who do
you think you are ? " we do not expect a
reply. The answer is a unicorn. His idea
of himself is fabulous, far too great to be
divulged, too infinitely important to be
exposed to the remotest risk of derogation
or satire. He dare not even look at it too
closely himself.

This life-goal, this fantasy of what he
thinks he could be *if* things were not against
him, is not to be understood as if it were
ever the real end in view, or the focus of a
man's practical conduct of life. It has
usually very little relation to reality. Its
original usefulness was simply an inner and
subjective compensation for a feeling of
inferiority, and it has been fortified for the
same purpose ever since. It was never
intended for realization in the world.
Yet the influence of such an imagination
upon life is of paramount importance.

Its nature can best be understood by

reference to the ideas which Vaihinger has expounded in his " Philosophy of ' As If ' ". Adler acknowledges his indebtedness to Vaihinger's conception, which shows how all human knowledge, even that which we call the " exact sciences ", is based upon certain assumptions, which are taken thenceforth *as if* they were absolute truth. These assumptions are not recognized by us to be arbitrary, because they *work* as if they were absolute truth—unless and until we modify them by making another assumption. What we call a truth is in reality a " directive fiction ", and these directive fictions, meaningless in themselves, have the greatest importance in practice because we work by them. There is something in the psyche of the individual of this same nature—a directive fiction which is unacknowledged just because it is implicit in everything the individual thinks and does. It is this which determines the life-goal.

Life-goals are so very different in content, so individual, that we must beware of generalization in describing them. What is certainly common to them all is the idea or imagination of *superiority*. They are designed to balance some disadvantage, which has been felt as a tendency towards actual impotence, by giving oneself credit for some higher potentiality or even omnipotence. The existence of this mechanism can be traced by anyone with little trouble. In the course of almost any conversation between two persons (unless it is dominated wholly by a common objective interest), one may observe a continual if subtle effort of each to demonstrate some ascendency over the other. If one of them is made to feel in the inferior position he will immediately compensate by a thought of something in which he excels, perhaps quite unrelated to the subject of conversation, but which he will very likely drag into it. Failing that, he may make up for what he feels as a sort of defeat by thinking how good he is to bear it without retaliation—one of the most godlike of all assumptions of superiority.

These imaginations about himself, by means of which an individual balances his account with life, are all of some homogeneous character and make up the *directive fiction* of the life. They are a bundle of ideas about his own disadvantages, united with corresponding ideas of how to gain advantages. This bundle of ideas of advantage and disadvantage is the real centre of the individuality itself, to which everything else gets related. Quite individual and unique as it is in every case, it always acts as a striving from *below to above*. If we trace it from its beginning, it follows the usual course of development of directive fictions. Vaihinger says that the directive fiction, which begins as a pure fiction, is next taken as a hypothesis, at which stage it confirms itself, for whatever it may be it will be possible to amass experience which confirms it. Finally it is established as the dogma, when it still has directive usefulness, but begins to wage futile war with reality.

Thus the child's sense of inferiority, that he is small, weak, neglected or whatever other grievance may loom largest in his little world, is compensated by the consoling *fiction* that there is a " godlike " state of supremacy and domination to be attained—the more severe the former, the more fantastic will be the latter. This gives rise, always more or less unconsciously, to the *hypothesis* that all others and the world are keeping him out of his right, are *against* him. The very existence of such a hypothesis naturally modifies the attitude to life in such a way as to antagonize others and bring about confirmation, over and above the usual inclemency of life. The stage of *dogma* is soon reached, when the world and society are instinctively and constantly felt as hostile to his real interests, and the soul becomes fixedly oriented towards a goal of secure and isolated supremacy. This is, of course, the general outline of the development of the life-goal, even when the way to domination is sought by passive means, with more or less conscious notions of " overcoming through love ". In that case, what the individual understands by love is itself a roundabout way of possession, control or domination.

The formation of the life-goal takes place under the direction of what is called a *scheme of apperception*. This is simply to say that the individual perceives what he wants to perceive, and sifts out of his whole experience exactly what is useful in view of his directive fiction, forgetting or rejecting the rest of reality. In some cases, activities in the home or in the surroundings in which a child does not happen to be included are interpreted as proofs that he is slighted or not wanted. Of no importance in themselves, these things are noted with intense attention by the child, because they fit in with his scheme, they are evidence for the hypothesis he has already formed about life and which he is living solely to prove. Just as he thought, he must be very careful to attract attention. At a later stage of development, the same person will only display interest in the world according to the same scheme, noting how certain individuals attain power and others fail to do so. Such a psychic attitude may generally be inferred in the case of those people who show a strong interest in a world-figure such as Cæsar, Napoleon, or Mussolini or some other dictatorial personality, who symbolizes for them the way of attaining isolation, supremacy, and a sort of godlike irresponsibility, an ideal projection of their own striving. Those whose notion

c

of power is something magnetic, achieved through submission, will develop a fixed admiration for saints and great world-forsakers.

Individuality itself, in the human sense, depends upon this fact that there is always inferiority, against which a goal of superiority is erected. It is our salvation from living according to the mere instinct of the herd. Without his directive fiction, a man would simply not know what to do with himself and would fall under the totally unconscious sway of his biological destiny. He would still compensate for his actual organic inferiorities, in a real, but not in a human way. The human compensation is essentially through an idea because man has an idea of himself. It is when the idea of himself is, by his power of comparison, felt as subject to some sort of limitation or curtailment that it imperatively demands a corresponding idea of his freedom or aggrandisement.

This constant striving from below to above in the soul of man is precisely the same in the healthy and in the neurotic, for it is the basis of all individual orientation.

THE LIFE GOAL

What distinguishes the healthy is the greater strength of the communal feeling, which compels them to realize their desire for ascendency in more or less useful and realistic activities. The neurotic, on the other hand, is too seriously discouraged to believe in any power of realization, and thus intensifies the actual and practical inferiority of his position by inability to work, to make friends, or to face difficulties: all of which he compensates by attempting to regain, fantastically, the subjective *sense* of worth and potency. There is no perfectly healthy mind; but if there were, it would be maintained by such a strong interest in communal causes and needs, that there would be no time left for rumination upon personal deficiencies or failures, which would only be noticed in order to correct them as practically as possible in the immediate moment.

Such perfect mental health is attainable in theory at least and to a very high degree in practice, but the fact of human individuality is that it has always been lost before it is found. Adler's description of the life-goal explains the nature of the fact, which is known to every good intuitive psychologist, that the inner tension of any personality (his sense of distance from his own ideal) is closely related to the tensions he creates in his society. His hostility to his environment originates together with the subjective or " godlike " ambition, as part of the same process. The inner tension is caused by the incompatibility of such an ambition with the obvious reality of the individual's conduct : so that he divides himself into a " higher " and " lower " nature, associating his true self with the former and rejecting the latter as " not-self ", as the obstacle to perfect action and therefore the excuse for impotence. He artificially splits up his personality and regards certain impulses as outside his control, thus washing his hands of responsibility for them. They are " in him ", but not himself. We can see the beginnings of the process in a child who was reproved for picking his nose and answered: " I don't want to do it, but my hand does ".

When religion enters the life, it often plays upon this primordial fantasy and intensifies it—generally and properly with the object of increasing the communal element in the " higher self ", but all too frequently the effect is only to strengthen the soul's reliance upon " its own God ", which heightens the will to power and withdraws the devotee more firmly from any realities except those which sustain him in the "holy of holies", which may be the vague sense of a splendour of being, a potentiality which he never believes in as actuality. Religion is now outwitted by the greater intelligence and subtlety of the modern soul, which can all too easily use it as a means to its neurotic goals. A training in Individual Psychology must be considered indispensable to the ministry of religion.

Whatever value they may have in certain systems of philosophy, the conceptions of " higher " and " lower " nature are found, in Individual Psychology, to be generally tricks of apperception, in the service of a single and unified life-plan. The life-plan is the *entire system of behaviour* by means of which the individual keeps, secure and inaccessible, his superiority from the test of reality. What are called " lower " tendencies are among those tricks of behaviour no less than many of the good words and works of the same person. If he did not prove to himself that he is unworthy of his goal, he would have to attempt to realize it, in which case he suspects he might lose it. His assertion of his own immoral tendencies thus plays the part of a " certificate of illness ", excusing his non-realization. Let us repeat that the directive fiction was never designed for realization although it is of an apparently realizable nature. Its purpose is the heightening of the ego-feeling by an inner assurance of worth, and as such it is the sacred stronghold of the individuality. The more a man gains practical recognition for his work and achievement, of course, the less he is really dependent upon his subjective compensation, but he never gives it up. The healthy man, however, does not have to waste most of his energy in safeguarding it, like the neurotic.

This conception of the life-goal as the fictitious principle of individuality is the central idea of Individual Psychology, and that which provokes the greatest opposition. The resistance which many oppose to it is personal, for they feel that it threatens their own self-valuation, and calls their life-goals into question. But there are others who object more reasonably to the idea that individuality can be founded upon a sense of defect and inferiority. They point out that the sense of oneself as " godlike "—a word which Dr Adler uses in an almost satirical sense in speaking of the neurotic ambition—is often a recognition of certain supreme values, ethical or æsthetic, and they object to deriving these values from mere deficiency.

These critics must examine the facts more closely. It is true that the personality-ideal, which it is the goal of life to preserve, is very often harmonized with certain moral ideas which improve the relation to life so far as they are verified in practice. But the modern physician and psychiatrist are faced with the fact that many patients, and others who are on the way to become patients, are persons who, in spite of amiable traits of character, high ideals and even social usefulness, are suffering from emotional disturbance, obsessions and moral disintegration. Whatever valuable elements we may discern in the life-line of one of these, it is obviously impractical as a whole. As a whole, moreover, we can see how both moral and immoral elements fall into line in the tendency towards a certain kind of superiority. The subject is trying to redress a balance—to compensate, with a permanent sense of failure to do so completely. This is but an intensification of the state in which the modern soul lives normally.

The ideal elements in the life-goal are often the surest clue to its fantastic character. If asked: " What do you really want to become ? " the reply of the neurotic would generally include the possession of certain virtues, such as courage, truthfulness or universal love. An impartial examination of the conduct of the life would however show, in nearly every case, a notable deficiency in the exercise of the valued virtue, in spite of the subject's strange efforts to prove to himself that he possessed it. The attitude is of course unrealistic. The idea of *possessing* a virtue is in itself inconsistent, since virtues are essentially the constant qualities of a person's entire conduct in relation to all others. Apart from this reality in exercise, the conception of possessing the virtue is only a heightening of the sense of one's own *separate* value. The effect of this is to diminish the value of life and society, giving a sense of futility to the real everyday existence, which has to be compensated by a further effort at self-exaltation, thus completing the vicious circle.

The life-goal is such that the individual can give no reliable or satisfactory account of it, even if he is not particularly neurotic. It seems to have this abstract quality of *being* rather than *doing*, is rationalized somewhat vaguely and heroically, so that Adler constantly refers to it as " ambitious ". It is only by a high degree of very objective self-observation and introspection, which is exceedingly rare, that any individual can distinguish it as the constellation of guiding motives which it really is. The self-observation required is purely scientific in spirit, equally free from partiality and vindictiveness : for an attitude of self-condemnation is a certain sign of attachment to an ideal self-valuation, and mobilizes all the forces of compensation. In most cases where it has become necessary for a man to recognize the true nature of his goal, it is only possible with the aid of the physician's encouragement and skill.

Almost any of Dr Adler's published cases can be taken to illustrate the difficulty. One of them relates how a man who had been brought up in great disharmony with a widowed mother, became engaged to a girl of high character, and very curiously failed in the engagement. He began to put his *fiancée* through severe tests. He was an unusually gifted and refined personality, and he required her to educate herself in accordance with his own ideal of culture. He pushed this tutorial attitude to the point where she finally rebelled and broke the engagement, upon which he had a nervous breakdown and became incapable of work.

Analysis revealed the idea which this man had formed concerning women, principally from experience of his mother's influence. He had a sense of inferiority, of a lack of virility, and believed he would never be able to dominate a woman. It is noteworthy that domination had become indispensable to his idea of a happy relation with a woman! Above all things, it seemed necessary to him to escape subordination to the female, to achieve a superiority in that particular relation. That was why he tried to force his beloved into his own special line of activity where he would be master. When even this did not promise absolutely certain supremacy, he provoked a situation which would enable him to escape altogether.

The subsequent breakdown was the man's final vindication of his fantastic ideal. It followed, as is usual, the pattern of his childish rebellions, when he had refused to eat, sleep, or to do anything, and had behaved as though seriously ill. Now he had an illness which impaired his entire fitness for life, and the woman was responsible for it! He had reached the superior position in both culture and character. By this last desperate device, moreover, he had given himself an experience which would protect him against marriage for the rest of his life.

It would be obviously impossible for such a man to admit to himself : " I want to achieve absolute supremacy and independence in regard to woman ". His culture and his communal feeling prohibit such an idea. Nevertheless, such is the need of his being—a need growing out of his whole past, and even grafted on to biological roots. He works to realize it, not objectively, by conscious work, which in any case would be impossible—but subjectively, by an elaborate *détour*, by an arrangement of his experiences and his emotions. He must continue to do this to the end, whatever the practical disadvantage, unless he can become conscious of what he is doing. To detect the nature of such a case, or indeed to penetrate the mystery of any individual's style of life, we have to make a synthetic picture of his strivings, observing the conditions he is succeeding in establishing both in his own thought and in his environment. It then appears exactly *as if* he were straining towards a certain imagined goal, an appearance which is soon verified as the most comprehensive and useful truth about him.

The purpose of Individual Psychology is to divine the unconscious life-goal, when it threatens the conscious purpose and realization of the individual. It aims therefore at a complete portrait of the personality. The first appearance of the man, his manner and social bearing, his position in the family, his characteristic postures, the nature of his thoughts in success and failure—all are studied as organically related in a dominant tendency to achieve something. Almost any impartial observer of intelligence, it may be said, thus confronted with a comprehensive account of a man's style of life, would be likely to divine its guiding fiction considerably better than the man himself. But a true psychological diagnosis needs the gift of *empathy*—that is, it requires the power of entering into another's experience as if it were one's own, which results in something much more like the presentation of an artist than the description of a scientist. The gift of empathy, rare as it is, is achieved

THE LIFE GOAL

by all whose own goal of life has been transformed by a true consciousness of its guiding fiction. That is, as it has always been, the high human value of the repentant sinner.

CHAPTER III

PSYCHOLOGY AND SOCIAL SCIENCE

THE discoveries of psycho-analysis are such that their effect cannot be limited to the practice of doctors or confined to the experiences of patients. They alter our view of human nature in a way which is bound to affect our beliefs concerning the family, the relations of the sexes, and even property and law.

Considered even as a purely medical procedure, the new psychology is a practice in which society as a whole has an interest. The nervous diseases, which in the modern world have assumed the proportions of a plague, are not like ordinary illnesses. They are not caught nor inherited nor contracted in the manner of most diseases ; but, as has been amply proved, they are really self-inflicted. That is as much as to say that they are diseases of the will and it is impossible to regard aberrations of the will, or the way in which we treat them, in isolation from ethics and the community.

The fury of opposition which was aroused by the Freudian publications is thus very intelligible. Freud's theory of the Neuroses, in the way in which it was presented, opened up a vista of alarming social possibilities. It ascribed the plague which is disabling modern civilization entirely to sexual repression. Freud himself has always been far from imagining that this plague could be cured by a social policy of unlimited sexuality. The most elementary psychologist, much more a master like Freud, is in no danger of confusing repression with abstinence, or sensuality with sanity. A public victory for the Freudian views, however, would certainly not bring about the accurate understanding of them; and it could hardly fail to be taken by the uninitiated as an authorization of almost promiscuous relations. Many modern idealists of undoubted honesty, socialist and otherwise, have believed in a larger liberation of the sexual life, and there was much to be said for it even before Freud;

but the hardiest revolutionary would be nervous at the prospect of a re-organization of Society upon the basis of sexual hygiene alone especially as Freud has not given us the smallest notion how to do it.

Apart from all superficial misunderstandings of his writings, Freud does give the impression that sex is the most misunderstood of all forces and that its expression is the central problem of life. He is bent upon demonstrating, not only from pathology, but from his marvellously acute observation of everyday life, that every activity of both individual and social existence is woven into the sexual striving and tinctured by it. It appears as if all human life, from the cradle to the grave, is really dominated and shaped by the longing for sexual union. His work as a whole is a formidable argument that the firm regulation of sex by society is an evil, and that civilization is, in an essential way, contrary to man's nature.

It is difficult, upon purely scientific grounds, to forgive Freud for the onesided character of his hypothesis. He must have known, by the elementary facts of biology,

D

that there is a grave objection to founding a psychology upon the will to conjugation, for a thinker of Freud's calibre does not ignore the light which the sciences reflect upon each other.   If his theory were justifiable we should find the fact of conjugation not only central but absolutely dominant throughout the realm of biology, and especially in the lowest and most primitive forms of life.   But what do we really find?   The most primitive kind of generation, and almost certainly its orignal form, is effected without conjugation at all, by simple budding or fission.   The cell divides into two halves, each of which grows into a whole, and far from losing by the process, it is not only doubled but, to a certain extent, rejuvenated by it.   With most organisms of one cell only, however, the reverse process is also necessary to reinvigorate their life ;   and they conjugate—that is, two cells make a contact and coalesce perfectly to form a single cell, which afterwards proceeds to further divisions.   The process of *growth* in all organisms of more than one cell is accomplished by division, the re-duplicated cells remaining adjacent instead of separating one from another. Millions of further generations take place without any more conjugation—at any rate, in the sense of coalescence.

Now the single cell is the biological unit, a thing with a measure of independent existence, the molecule, as it were, of organic being ; and it would be unreasonable to suppose that it is not also in some sort the representative psychic unit. And it is evident that its psychic orientation cannot be wholly towards conjugation. The opposite process, of fission, must have its psychic counterpart, although we cannot find it in Freud's psychology. The multi-cellular organism, the chief glory of creation, grows to perfection by the ceaseless division and differentiation of its component cells. The minimum of conjugation and the maximum of division goes to its making. It is made possible, indeed, because its myriads of beings cut themselves off and adventure into independence, not because they all coalesce into an unity.[1] From

[1] Compare with this the *Hostile Symbiosis* of Morley Roberts.

these premises of biology alone, we should naturally expect that the impulse towards individuation and separate existence is indeed more primordial, more inherent in life itself, than the impulse towards union, which latter indeed appears more like a device of which the individuality avails itself.

A purely sexual psychology, therefore, is not only socially impracticable but biologically eccentric. As an instrument of practical psycho-therapy it must be admitted to have had great, although limited, usefulness : but, properly understood, its social implications are not so much evil as intangible. You cannot found any structure upon the human relationship which is *par excellence* the most shifting and elusive in its nature. The historical and indispensable institution of the family is certainly not founded upon sexual expression or even hygiene as Freud understands these things. However highly we may value perfection of the erotic life, it appears to be more like the added grace of a higher culture than in any sense its basis. On the other hand, the will to self-existence, which for Adler is the root-principle of the psyche, is also central in the social life, of which it is both the problem and the solution. Egoism is always at the root of social difficulties, on the one hand ; and, on the other, it is original and self-affirmative personalities who give life to the community.

The immense social value of Adler's work is in its detection of the strict correspondence between sanity and social orientation, so that we see the soul's integrity and happiness as features of its social functioning. This is not a new truth. Its verification through analytical psychology is, however, a new and much-needed service to our times. In this age of excessive individualism even religion has lost most of its ancient power to demonstrate this truth, and we have seen religion itself infected by the prevailing spirit—becoming highly " personal ", patriotic and even class-conscious. While religion of this kind retains some power of external discipline, it loses most of its power to harmonize the psychic life, and represses the individual more than it liberates him. Religious ideas such as Heaven and sin and Hell, which are no longer believed in as external realities can, however, be rediscovered as internal facts through Individual Psychology, and individuality itself can be detected clearly as the fall of man, from which he is saved only by the attainment of usefulness.

Although no one could call Adler an optimist, his system of Individual Psychology is founded upon encouragement, and is deeply reassuring. For while it reveals evil in our most intimate aspirations and idealistic fantasies, with a probe too searching for any soul to elude, it reveals also the function of evil in the human kingdom, and the way of its continual redemption. It shows that the sins of the individual are in truth no more purely *his own* than are his virtues : by imagining that he owns his virtue he cannot escape thinking that he owns also his sins, and it is largely that which puts him in their power. And it points a way out of both his imagined guilt and fantastic innocence, by showing how real power and usefulness can be educed from the life-plan which was formed as an escape from reality and a vantage ground against the world.

Adler's standpoint is " beyond good and evil " in the Nietzchean sense, for the utmost affirmation of personality may be psychologically sound so long as it is made in the common interest. The will to heighten the sense of individual being is ineradicable, and no social progress, no creation of general interest and no development would be possible without it. The need of society is for self-reliant and autonomous individuals, whose self-assertion is balanced by communal feeling and intelligence, but not inhibited by communal restraints which only cause feelings of inferiority. It is right and natural that everyone should love human society and culture, which are the source of his entire human being and the only sane objects of his activity, but we must recognize that human organization is very imperfect. It drives many into a concealed or open revolt against it, and ultimately into a despair of being able to do anything with their lives. Yet this very imperfection of human social organization is really the open door and the opportunity of useful power for every human soul.

Once given the feeling of inferiority in social relations, it is impossible that a soul should not make some compensation, and it is quite likely to be of a socially useless nature. Alcoholism and sensuality generally are to be understood in this way. The usual effect of alcohol and of sexuality is to restore the lowered sense of personal existence to lofty heights, where the psyche is enthroned in a kingdom of vague subjective opulence which cannot be shared with anyone. These things, which appear outwardly as mere sensuality, are from the victim's own point of view highly spiritual compensations for a feeling of frustrated ambition; though of course they intensify the evil by making a man more ashamed and hopeless than ever in contact with the real world.

But there are more positive compensations for the sense of social impotence. Socialism is an example of such a compensation which has an intelligible and communal aim. When the peasantry of Western Europe became the wage-earners of

industrial life, they felt, as a class, excommu-
nicated. They had become the instruments
instead of the members of a society, a
subordinate class whose relation with
the rest was now liquidated by a mere
exchange of money and service. They
became " class-conscious ", as they called
it, and repudiated all debt to the civilization
in which they found themselves. At the
same time they produced, in compensation
for the social expression they lacked, the
vision of Communism. Their efforts to
impose this vision upon the world are of
great historic importance and are leading
to drastic changes in social life. We may
leave out of account the relative value
of Communism among the political movements of our time. From the standpoint
of the psychologist all political movements
may be good, so far as they direct the
interest and intelligence towards communal
questions and needs. But if we take
Communism, for the moment, as a collective
fantasy, a dream of a golden age in the
future, we are bound also to recognize that
any class of men, in such a position of
inferiority as the proletariat, would

necessarily produce such a directive fiction. In accordance with the same psychological law, the Jews compensate for their national weakness and dispersion by the most flamboyantly nationalistic of all religions, and exceed the world-influence of any nation of their size by their extraordinary self-assertiveness in affairs.

It is the outcasts whose will to power is the most irresistible. It is not by chance that the World-Transformer of the Christian Mystery was born in a stable. The forces of social revolution, of social fantasy aspiring to overthrow and supplant the existing empire of the world, are supplied either by disinherited classes of men, or by intellectuals with a deep and bitter sense of being excluded by the society they live in. A leading part in such activity is also taken by those whose position in the family intensifies the inferior feelings of childhood. Adler claims that a large proportion of those men who have risen from obscure beginnings to places of eminence and power have been youngest children, and the youngest of the family is usually the most restless and ambitious nature.   In the army Adler was generally able to distinguish the last-born children, merely by their bearing on parade.

All positions of inferiority, whether due to family, social or individual experience, find compensation in the pattern of a man's life-plan, even when he is working it out with a sane outlook and a good social direction.   Failures occur when the individual feels unable to attain to any practical superiority and becomes quite discouraged. Nothing seems left for him to do but to withdraw from the demands of society and take his own way.   This being, in reality, impossible for a man to do—and even absurd in idea—he does not acknowledge the desire, but adopts a style of life which secures the necessary advantages of society, as far as possible, while evading the demands. To do this, without *lèse majesté* to his ego-ideal, often requires the most astonishing détours :   such, for example, as adopting a compulsion neurosis.   A person with a compulsion really believes that he is obliged, by a power greater than himself, to do certain entirely useless, fanciful or even disgusting things.   He thus gets into a state of distress, inner complication and general disability which effectively removes him from normal social demands; and, strange to say, all the suffering is worth while to him, because he triumphs over the compulsion of his environment. Society has been resisted and beaten, however miserable the victor may be. He cannot however, rejoice in his victory; he must not even know it too clearly, or the childish nature of it would become at once apparent to him.

But it is not only these extreme cases of complete breakdown that reveal the sense of inferiority compensated by withdrawal into psychic isolation. There are able men, capable of working well and even of filling high positions of responsibility, whose activities are in reality but devices of safety, calculated to protect them from any real community of life with others. In some cases the main motive of their work is to evade more intimate responsibility. A fixed desire to accumulate money, for example, is in itself a means of attaining irresponsible power. A miserly and grasping tendency, often well camouflaged, is developed in order to be safe against the social environment, which is felt as if it were something mercilessly hostile. There are also instances of immoderate overwork, without any parsimony or covetousness, which are clearly traceable to the determination to achieve through industry an irreproachable position—which is also, by the way, an unapproachable one, as in the too familiar cases of women who degenerate into disagreeable but highly efficient housewives. These must be counted as examples of psychic disease, in spite of a limited amount of social adaptation and usefulness, for the personality is really developing in opposition to the community under cover of a service which is, in the last analysis, not genuine. Such are the hard-faced and self-righteous men, the spuriousness of whose social service can often be traced in its effects, for it is their spirit in business, law, politics and affairs generally which hardens the temper of public life under a meretricious appearance of efficiency, and on the whole it drives the state towards war and revolution.

It is chiefly from these aberrations of the

will that Individual Psychology has been
able to demonstrate the nature of it, to
show that the psyche is but the instrument
of the will to superiority, the will to remedy
one's weakness in the face of Nature and
Society. But the same investigation has
shown also what is its norm : its way to
realization and the peace of fulfilment.
Since the sickness of the mind can be traced
to its illusion of isolation, to its loss of
social courage and communication, we can
see the condition of its cure. The psyche
itself is indeed hard to change, but an
individual can adopt a different attitude
towards himself, not by introspection, with
its further self-concentration, so much as
by giving due weight to the attitude of
others towards him. He can regain
consciously the communal interest which
he has unconsciously lost. This demands the
sacrifice of the irrational striving for power
which he has developed. But, in so far as
he does this, real power descends unsought
upon him, for he is one with his community
and naturally a power within it. He has
the natural weight and influence of one
whose service is real. Not that this feels

like power : nor is it exercised with any relish of domination. It feels like peace, for it is the true goal of the will and the right compensation for the weakness of individual existence.

The healthy social outlook implied by Individual Psychology has in some quarters proved to be anything but a recommendation. It is suspected that such a psychology is not a science, but only an ethical system in scientific disguise. Such a suspicion is easy to understand, but it is quite mistaken. Dr Alexander Neuer has convincingly shown that psychology is gaining a basis of equality with the other sciences for the first time since Adler's contribution. And this not only because it is biologically based, but because it is socially conceived.

It is the human mind which is the subject of psychology, and the distinctive quality of the human mind is the quality of its intelligence, which is conditioned by language. Language is not an individual creation, but essentially the co-operative production of all men since the beginning of their history. The intelligence of the individual, his actual power of thinking in words, is the work of the human race. The psychologist, it is true, is not interested in the thinking processes alone. He looks for the will which animates the thinking. But since he is studying man and not the rhinoceros, he is bound to relate every emotional state to the kind of thinking with which it is associated.

Freud's great innovation in psycho-therapeutic technique was to make the patient develop his thoughts aloud by what is called " free association "—which means putting one's thoughts into words continuously and openly as they occur. By the way in which a man carries out this difficult exercise the psychologist can see which thoughts are the most involved with emotions. He can detect the " resistances " by the ideas which the subject cannot put into words without emotional stress, and note those which he expresses with ease and pleasure. But why does the man talk to himself at all? Why does a flow of words so usually accompany the succession of images and pictures that flit through the soul, whether alone or in company with others? There is but one reasonable explanation. The individual is ceaselessly striving to assert his own nature upon the level of human intelligibility, to exhibit himself, even if only *to* himself, *sub specie humanitatis*. To translate any emotional striving into language is to render it, potentially at all events, a communicable human thought. It is true that the thinker often has no intention of speaking his thought to a single other soul, which makes it all the more remarkable that he should put it into intelligible form. Evidently intelligibility is an end in itself as well as a means to the mastery of the environment. The fundamental striving of the soul for self-existence demands this. The individual must feel himself to be a being with *meaning*, for he cannot have human importance without it. Hence if he does not explain himself to others he does so to himself, or perhaps imagines that he does it, for much internal talking is of a very shabby quality.

Early in his work, Freud was struck by the fact that the most painful emotional states were relieved, as if by magic, at the moment that the patient could correctly account for them. He must also have observed that even an incorrect explanation, if logically complete and credible, is a temporary island of refuge for the soul. What emerges with certainty is that the will, whatever hypothesis we may have as to its essential nature, is pacified and released by the attainment of intelligibility. Beyond this fact little or nothing has been established, by all the labours of psycho-analysis, which could be called 'scientific' in the strictly modern and inductive sense ; excepting only the striving for supremacy. And it is not difficult to see that these two are one. For an individual, placed in any position of inferiority, can escape the hopeless *feeling* of inferiority if he can formulate the situation. By the formulation he not only becomes in a certain sense *equal* to it, but also feels that he achieves a kind of unity with the rest of mankind : he establishes a communication, potential if not actual. That sense of being in communication may be called the norm of psychic health. It has of course nothing to do with the sense of being in conventionally correct relation with others. On the contrary, the acceptance of the conventions of gregarious life, if they are taken as something absolute and not merely instrumental, is an attempt to short-circuit the life-process of attaining intelligibility by a rough formulation imposed once and for all. The purely conventional man, if for the moment we may set up such an abstraction, feeling that the hostility of souls to each other makes spontaneous understanding impossible, tries to base his understanding of his relation to the community upon social custom alone. Since a large part of his reality cannot possibly be so understood, his striving for intelligibility is chiefly turned into unconscious struggle for power, with the inevitable tendency to neurosis. It is necessary to mental health that we should feel free to reformulate the situation *as a whole* at any moment. So long as the soul feels that it is moving towards intelligibility no other kind of privation can fatally affect its health.

It may, of course, be asked whether this conception of the human will as fixed towards the attainment of power and intelligibility can be taken as anything more than theory. If

Freud's hypothesis of the will as essentially will to conjugation is only hypothesis and no more, can we claim for Adler's theory any greater certainty? The answer is one which would apply to any kind of scientific generalization. The only possible instrument of thought by which we can grasp the experimental facts of any subject is its theory, or hypothesis. As explained above, it is a tendency of the mind, strengthened by training, to translate experience into human meaning, which we do by the use of concepts, or in the case of more extended experiences by theories. The theory, as Vaihinger has demonstrated, is no better than a fiction in relation to reality, but it gives us a way of approach to reality. It not only gives us this practical advantage, but also colours and bends the world to our vision, for it makes us both act and perceive things exactly "as if" it were the final truth about them. Either implicitly or explicitly we are always living by a hypothesis. Even the most universally-used principles of mathematics and of logic have this fictional foundation, since there is no escape from this human dilemma—that the absolute truth is not known to us, but we must nevertheless act as if it were.

In the original choice of our fiction (apart from the particular nature of the need for it), there is something entirely free and optional. In this matter of psychology we are free to imagine the human mind as inflexibly oriented towards individual sexual expression. On the other hand, we are free to conceive it as bent upon compensating its own insufficiency by power in the community—an idea which it often perverts into that of power *against* the community. The adoption of neither of these views will endow us with omniscience of reality, but both are potent to create an entire view of life. Moreover, men create their life anew according to their view of it.

But which, it may be insisted, is the more likely to be the truth? Is the heart of man, the secret striving of his soul, directed more towards the womb or to the world? Is it towards the emotions of coalescence or towards the intelligible splendours of individuality and culture?

The findings of psychology, since Adler, tend decidedly towards the latter view. But let it be granted that facts are not final proof, since all the facts can never be known. And whoever the investigator may be, he also started with his guiding fiction, he has his scheme of apperception. Knowing this, Adler has not concealed his own choice, he has made no attempt to play upon the false magic of the word " science " as it is commonly misunderstood by the ignorant. Here is his declaration—

" We cannot escape from the net of our own relatedness. Our sole safety is to assume the logic of our communal existence upon this planet as an *ultimate absolute truth*, which we approach, step by step, through the conquest of illusions arising from our incomplete organization and limited capabilities as human beings."

Granting that assumption, the sole assumption possible under the circumstances, a science of Individual Psychology can be founded upon a reasonable and even impregnable basis. It is this which

Adler has done by showing that all psycho-pathology is of the nature of egoism. Egoism in all its innumerable forms is the attempt of the individual to compensate for an illusory loss of individuality.

The discoveries of Individual Psychology do not contradict those of psycho-analysis in general, as to the existence of sexual complications in all forms of psychic ill-health. They decidedly confirm the importance of a sound and normal love-life, which however is the result of a progressive individual power in social usefulness. Individual Psychology is not an escape from Freud's gloomy diagnosis of the modern soul. It rather increases the terror of our predicament, for it shows a deeper danger in man than his sensuality. The dragon is still more fearful than the slime. If Freud has exposed the beast in man, it is Adler who has revealed the devil.

CHAPTER IV

MAN AND WOMAN

There have been innumerable attempts to explain the difference between the souls of man and woman. These attempts, which range from ingenuity to genius have not, however, provided humanity with any useful working truth about the sexes which could strengthen their co-operation or make them happier. On the whole, they have had just the opposite effect. For the most part they have been efforts to prove some difference of an abstract, absolute kind between the male and female natures. In such writings as those of Schopenhauer, Nietzsche and Weininger upon woman, we find the sexes antithesized, as though their fundamental natures were poles asunder, and in cosmic opposition. This antithesizing of the sexes in thought tends to antagonize them in imagination and in reality. On the other hand the work

[72]

of an artist such as Dostoievsky or Shakespeare differentiates man from woman, but it also unites them in the same human reality, which we share through the same gift of empathy.

All efforts to sum up maleness and femaleness in absolute concepts tend towards the kind of conclusion that Weininger reached in *Sex and Character*. In that work of genius it was proved, with great force and plausibility, that man and woman are really in a kind of pure logical opposition, like all and nothing, or being and non-being, infinity and zero. Hence, it is to man that the power and glory of life belongs, to woman the submission and the ignominy. Man is pure will and intelligence, and woman blind instinct and trickery, if we could analyse them both to their depths. Weininger softened the harshness of this distinction by saying that there was no such thing as an absolutely male man or an absolutely female woman. There were only all degrees of mixture predominating one way or the other ; and, ultimately, the only way to reform woman was to treat her as if she were man.

MAN AND WOMAN

Now this tendency to philosophize about the sexes until they appear to be the Yea and Nay of the Absolute, of which Weininger is the supreme exponent, is an expression of a general human failing, a habit of thinking of man as *above* and woman as *below* in the order of human value. Prevalent and ancient as it is, this habit of thought is a vital factor in the psyche. The movements of feminism, which have revolted against it, have been unable to free themselves entirely from it. They too often betray a note of protest, by an effort to turn the tables, as in the case of learned feminists who have urged that the female is much the more important in nature, where the male has often a very temporary and instrumental existence, dwindling in some species to that of a mere minute parasite upon the female. They have also made much of the idea that human society originated in matriarchy, in the rule of women. These original theses have shown that it is possible to construct a good contrary argument, but the important fact for the psychologists is that the notion of masculinity as something privileged and

superior is what we find in every psyche,
male or female, and that, the more neurotic
the soul, the more it instinctively conceives
femaleness as a degradation and maleness
as an ideal.

To Adler the question is not " Is man, in
cosmic truth, a higher order of being than
woman ? "—a question he would think idle
and purposeless in itself—but " *Why* do
we think there is a superiority in maleness,
and *what effect* does the idea have on our
lives ? " The idea has no inherent or a
priori necessity, yet it is so widespread, as
an unconscious assumption, that it may be
said to be universal. That it is so is verified
by the intimate investigation of psycho-
analysts, which only confirms the observations
of most intuitive observers.

The idea of femininity itself is associated
with feelings of inferiority, frequently from
early days of childhood. We find that a
small boy, asked temporarily to wear a
girl's garment, or to assume one he regards
as girlish, may respond with an unexpected
fit of temper ; and a little later he may show
the same resistance to riding a girl's bicycle.
Girls, on the other hand, may take a delight

in boyish garb and boyish sport, such as football or climbing trees, obviously beyond the normal interest which such things might have for them. It is clear that in the upward striving of the ego, in its scheme of self-valuation, femininity has already been conceived as a position of inferiority to be avoided, and masculinity as a goal of superiority to be striven for.

This is largely accounted for by the profound impression made upon the child by the relative position of the adults around it, especially that of the father and mother. In the vast majority of cases the father, spending comparatively short intervals in the home, coming and going, and in contact with a wider and mysterious sphere, appears to stand for almost god-like qualities of domination and irresponsibility. The real inequality of privilege and freedom in father and mother, which is often great enough, is further magnified by the imperfection of the child's view of it. Nevertheless, it is the child's own sense of inferiority which fastens upon both the realities and the appearances of masculine superiority, and invests them with a sort of abstract absoluteness. Masculinity becomes an essential quality of the life-goal. Although this is mitigated to the extent that the feeling of community and unity prevails in the home life, the feeling of inferiority is in the experience of every child, as we have seen, and it is almost inevitable that it should be related to the distinction of sex.

In the experience of later life there is so much which strengthens the sense of antithesis between male and female that it becomes woven into the texture of thought itself. The very connotation of such words as "manly" "masculine" and "virile", in our common speech, includes the ideas of force, conquest, self-assertion and irresponsibility, while "feminine" or "womanly" are often used to connote actual inferiority; and at the best they include attractiveness and the passive virtues, but never any idea of power or domination. The fictive goal of glorious egoity which directs the upward strivings of the soul from its sense of inferiority is thus naturally conceived as masculine. In woman this leads to attempts to escape the feminine rôle in life, and in man to strange efforts to attain to some supermanliness.

Thus it is often found, in the analysis of dreams, that a man will symbolize a humiliation or degradation of which he stands in fear by an image of himself as a woman, a mother, or in some feminine occupation : whereas a woman is likely to dream of herself as a man when she is preparing herself in some way to triumph over her environment.

These conceptions of masculinity and femininity as higher and lower, or, still more abstractly, as polar opposites, positive and negative, are simply illusions due to the upward striving of individuals, the striving which makes them see every alternative in terms of absolute advantage or disadvantage. Such conceptions have no connection with the real and profound *difference* between man and woman. Their omnipresence in speech and literature is continually vitiating the relations between the sexes.

In a certain passage in *Paradise Lost*, obviously inspired by a statement of St Paul, there is the familiar line—

" He for God only, she for God in him."

The practical effect of such a thought

(for we are not concerned with its theological or philosophical meaning) upon a person with a feeling of inferiority—and that is upon everybody—is to increase the desire to be male. It pictures man as the mediator between God and woman—the semi-god-like being. Far from making woman worship man, such statements cause her to try to escape from the womanly position and, if possible, to *be* man. In the case of a man, it may lead to thoughts of union with God, but what it is sure to produce is a wish for distance from woman —and distance in an upward direction. All such fantasies about the nature of sex strengthen the idea from which they originated. Under their influence both man and woman tend to refuse normal sex union, man because it makes him feel only *equal* with woman, and woman simply because it makes her feel a woman—i.e. an inferior being. At the same time, in order to have proof of his maleness, the man tends either to an ascetic ideal, or to the ideal of Don Juan—either no women or all women— since *one* woman is, in the end, a position of partnership and equality. The woman, similarly, refuses marriage, or more likely cohabitation after marriage, as a protest, or she may aspire to promiscuity with the implicit idea that it is man-like. Investigations into the psychology of prostitution have shown that the dominant feeling among women who ply this trade is the desire to escape from the feminine rôle. It is a very crude and forcible way of registering the " masculine protest ".

The " masculine protest " is a technical term in Individual Psychology for this psychic attitude, which is simply the distorted apprehension of sex-differences caused by the striving for superiority. It is just as important in man as in women, and continually complicates the relations of the sexes with useless and really meaningless efforts to achieve the upper hand for its own sake, or to escape from domination. Almost the entire striving for superiority may become focussed in a masculine protest, which conditions the whole psychic development. When it takes an active form in women they try, from an early age, to usurp the male position. They are aggressive in manner, adopt definitely masculine habits or tricks of behaviour, and endeavour to domineer over everyone around them. Upon the theory that maleness and femaleness are mixed quantities in every individual, these mannish women would be explained by saying that they were nearing the point of equality between maleness and femaleness ; there have even been theories that the degrees of sex-differentiation depend upon the secretions of certain glands in the body. As a matter of fact we still know too little to be able to generalize safely about the action of these glands on the psychic constitution ; and such ideas are not necessary to the understanding of the masculine protest. We can see how it arises from a person's scheme of apperception.[1]

But there are other women who protest in covert ways, whose attitude is outwardly resigned. They achieve some esteem and influence by their resignation and worthiness, but they betray, by their clumsy and awkward behaviour to things and persons, that they dislike and resent their status. Something in the depths of their being is sulking, as it were, or behaving

[1] See page 32.

F

with a covert rudeness. These are often constant friends who are a constant trial and embarrassment. They appear to be doing everything wrongly with the best of intentions. Their mentality is often rather philosophic, and it must be admitted that they are often very good persons, who protest against an intolerable lot with passive resistance and some genuine communal feeling. The worst swindlers are the women who profess simply to accept inferiority for their sex, a position which gives them a certain degree of advantage over the egoism of men. Joining in the cry against women, they can claim a large amount of irresponsibility as the weaker sex, and in the last resort they throw all the real burden of life's responsibility upon their men-folk. These are women with unaccountable changes of mood, violent tantrums and Cleopatra-like ideals, who often achieve considerable importance in small circles of which they are the greatest nuisance.

The masculine protest in a man is just as unfortunate in its consequences. Many men have never fully recovered from an infantile doubt as to whether they were really male ;

and the experiences of childhood frequently create in the growing boy a fear of women, which is a definite feeling of sex-inferiority. Such a boy will infallibly revenge himself upon woman somehow or other, and the prevalent fiction about masculine superiority will foster his fantastic striving towards an ideal of masculinity. This ideal masculinity is invariably conceived as the possession by himself of freedom, love and power, which in this egoistic conception amounts simply to irresponsibility, the *conquest* of women or friends, and the surpassing or overthrowing of others. Since there are insuperable obstacles in the way of a direct approach to this ideal goal, a man always makes more or less complicated détours to attain it, both in his outward conduct, and his inner arrangements of thought and emotion, but his artificial masculinity will not escape the eye of any well-trained observer of human nature.

How can the masculine protest be cured? The question is an embarrassing one, for this false scheme of valuation is deeply embedded in our civilization, and it would be rash to hope for a speedy improvement.

MAN AND WOMAN

In feminist movements and in the idealistic over-valuation of woman—often of a pathological origin—there is much which only intensifies the evil. Adler himself hopes much from the growth of co-education, the partial failure of which he ascribes to the element of competition which still survives in many co-educational schools, and robs the experiment of its value. But the greatest hope lies in the possibility of a general advance in the study of human nature, which alone can demonstrate how the idea of man and woman as above and below originates in distorted and antisocial ambitions. It will also make it clear that man and woman are, from the only practical human standpoint, not only equal but identical. We have no alternative but to educate them with the same mathematics, the same languages and the same ethics as men. It is only in function that they are different as a class, for in any society sex must to a certain extent be taken into account in the division of labour.

The fact that woman feels bullied by man and that man feels a need to assert himself above woman, is but part of a tyranny universal in our civilization. For we are living in a phase of human evolution when instinct is hectored and domineered by intellect. Instinct in both men and women is, in our day more than ever before, thwarted and encumbered with the overgrowth of intellectual conceptions, which obscure reality much more than they give power over facts. The precise demonstration of how this happens would take us too far into philosophy. But the true balance between intellect and instinct can nevertheless be found, for we are still human beings. To find it, however, men and women must co-operate with an aim of perfect equality not in couples only, but in larger groups where the distortions of individual relations are corrected by others and the common truths can be revealed. In this way they can do the real work of modern psychology, which is to pierce through the tangle of our intellectual complexities to the instinctive needs which rule the fate of every individual. In this way also their egocentric intellectualization can be dissolved, and they can approach the true norm of human reason, which is valid for all.

Marriage, the practical and realistic solution of the sexual problem, is the common task of man and woman. Its possibility is due to the fact that there is not inherently any opposition between the communal feeling and the erotic aspirations. It is only when the erotic striving has become mixed with feelings of compensation for inferiority that it drives towards anti-social realizations, and a purely egoistic satisfaction ; and then man and woman, individually and collectively, become involved in a mutual struggle for power.

Only in this connection, so far as I know, does Adler speak of an " iron law ", and the psychologist in him appears unmistakably as the moralist. There are many who may think this attitude severe, and who would always champion the claims of the individual against the community in questions of sexual partnership. But Adler has found once and for all that the claim of the community is implicit within the individual soul. It is the law of our own psychic being, much more than that of society, which punishes our errors in love, often after too long an interval for us to trace the cause of our suffering. Shallow libertarianism and glib convention are equally confounded before this discovery of man's inner need of communal meaning in the most intimate attachments of his soul. This focusses, more clearly than anything else, the unity of the inner and outer crisis of modern life. The present disorder in the ideals and practice of marriage, however, is ominous for the future of humanity, involving as it does all that makes for physical and spiritual well-being. Those who know best our present state of disintegration will be the least inclined to resent the impression, which Adler gives, that we must pass through a phase of grim grappling with duty and humble obedience to reality before we shall be able to read the truth of love and marriage, yet indelible where alone it is written, in the depth of every soul.

CHAPTER V

The general tendency of recent psychological interpretation has been to strengthen the idea of emotion as decisive in the individual's life. In all neurotic and abnormal states the patient appears to be driven by emotions. Since emotions thus seem to be causal, it is natural that physicians should have taken the obviously scientific course of tracing the emotions to ulterior feelings and anterior events. The total reversal of this apparently commonsense method is perhaps the most original and revolutionary thing in Adler's work. Man is not driven by his emotions: on the contrary, he produces them in order to attain his goal. All our moods and emotional crises are really very cleverly and subtly manufactured in order to see us through the difficulties of circumstances without injury to the indispensable aim of the ego.

THE MANAGEMENT OF EMOTION

Common sense and daily experience give some support to this view : for although we know that there are storms of emotion in which we are " not ourselves " and seem to be frustrating our own ends, we can often see clearly enough that the moods of others, whether playful, morose, sarcastic or humorous, are devices by which they are accustomed to get their own way. What if the grand passions also should be no less engineered—should be only deeper ruses to attain more secret ambitions? Adler goes even further, and declares that not only emotions but many physical sensations are thus self-induced. Painful as they may be, they are useful to us. Adler himself long resisted the conclusion, to which the facts of his practice finally forced him, that such agonizing pains as trigeminal neuralgia could be simply inflicted by the patient upon himself. When such distressing sensations can be adopted as instrumental by the soul, how much more obedient the emotions must be ! We have thus, in Individual Psychology, the beginning of a new classification of the emotions, according to the nature of their usefulness to the ego in its upward striving.

[89]

THE MANAGEMENT OF EMOTION

At the same time, we must recognize that the emotional being of any individual has its own particular character : certain emotions are interwoven with certain memories, in such a way that the stimulation of each emotion evokes all its own overtones and reverberations in the life-history of the psyche. The psyche might be compared to a harp of many chords, but it is the player himself who has made it. He plays what he likes, yet the music is largely conditioned by what he chose before.

We will trace the bearing of this observation upon an imaginary case of a man who is developing a suicidal tendency. Smith has frequently noticed, when waiting for the train by which he travels to town, that the thought of throwing himself upon the rails occurs to him. There is no particular " affect," the thought just crosses his mind. It is in reality the faint recurrence of an event of his childhood which he does not clearly remember, but, as we shall see, it is also *something more*. Smith's present situation is one of great worry and tension. He is in strained relations with his wife and he is failing to put his back into his business. Upon one or two recent occasions this imagination occurring to him upon the railway platform has given him a definite sensation of fear. Now, on leaving his home one morning to go to the station, after a nasty domestic crisis, he passes a steam road-roller. The same idea, of throwing himself under it, floats into his consciousness. This, he decides in a flash, is really serious ; it has never happened before ; he must be going mad. He re-inforces the thought with such a fit of terror that he cannot trust himself upon the platform at the station until the train is already standing there. He is then too disturbed to work at his office and returns early : and, upon the return journey to his house he is afraid to take the road in which the steam roller is working, and goes by another way. By this time of course, his state of fear and distress is such that he cannot take interest in anything but his own condition and he becomes a patient.

Dramatic cure of such a case may result from a typical psycho-analysis. In this procedure the patient will be led to trace out the origin of his suicide fantasies until he can clearly recount the childish situation in which, rebuked and rebuffed by his parents after a failure at school, he consoled himself with a very emotional day-dream of killing himself. Finally, he cannot but recall the fact that this was a fantasy not only of entirely satisfactory revenge for his injury, but also of winning the attention, love and pity which he desired. This very recollection, which he resists to the utmost, is, if properly brought about, a highly emotional experience which is called " abre-action." It releases this particular tension of the psyche by living through the experience anew in the full light of adult consciousness. It is so effective that the patient can immediately walk past a steam road-roller without taking any particular notice of it, and thinking all the while of something else.

Such excellent results, which have been often obtained, may easily lend themselves to a misinterpretation. It may be supposed that this particular fantasy of death, originating in a childish tragedy, has at last succeeded in taking possession of the adult man, and in driving him to its actual realization. But if past fantasies had anything like such potency we should all be mad, and society would be an impossibility. What has really happened is that the individual faced with pressing difficulties and *determined not to change* his life-line, has reanimated this ancient fantasy in order to attain his present goal. It is his quite real, though unrealistic, idea of gaining power over his environment. Either he will work himself up to the point of actual *felo de se*, with its masochistic triumph of wreaking revenge upon his circle and winning its compassion at the same time, or else he will attain the same result, only less dramatically, by having a mysterious illness. This question of interpretation is vital, for if we overvalue the importance of resolving the infantile tensions we lose sight of the fact that an individual's real problems are always in the present. Even a very well-conducted inquiry into a man's past history will never do him half as much good as his own honest effort to do justice to his personal relationships and to the logical demands of society. Such an inquiry, indeed, such a digging up of the foundations, is only occasionally made necessary because of the proud and obstinate determination of individuals not to revise their life-goals in the light of present urgencies.

The source of sanity is not in the past, however beautifully it may be clarified and revalued. It lies in social vision, in the love for the world and society as one's own counterpart and field of action. This vision is logically one with a man's own life-goal, for it is the world as he would like to live in it, and he knows by the simplest common-sense that he has to share it with others. His own vision of its culture and civilization is the spiritual dynamic of his existence, and it is this which inspires him to a practical and conceivable ambition.

This source of human sanity has been unfortunately ignored by the psycho-analytic schools, with the absurd result that they have been unable to account for culture except as a compulsory substitute for something else. Thus, to Freud, the true goal of the soul is death, symbolized by the incestuous return to the womb ; and the work of man in civilization is only rendered possible because society forbids indulgence in a life of pure incest and auto-sexuality : so that the same pleasures must be obtained in disguised or " surrogate " form. All the highest activities of culture are really nothing but these disguises or " sublimations," as they are called, of the seven kinds of auto-erotic gratification. A sculptor, for instance, is only finding a socially possible substitute for sexual gratification by the anus ; and the man whose emotional need is for the pleasure of giving pain finds its symbolic realization in the art of surgery, or, more humbly, in the trade of butchery. The emotional needs, centred in the sexual, are the driving force of life, and no other power is available for the work of human life. Thus we have a most perverse view, in which all the highest functions of mankind are reduced to the position of second-best substitutes for the lowest.

To anyone with a normal social vision such a view of the origin of culture not only seems repugnant—which it is—but also absurd, which is not altogether the case. It is true enough that the sculptor, so far as he fails in plastic vision, tends towards his own specific regression, which is likely to be of the order of anal-erotism, with its sensations of the moulding and modelling of material substance ; and the surgeon, to the extent that he is dissatisfied with his achievement or with the world's recognition of it, is more liable to revert to sadism than to any other perversion. But these emotional infantilities, far from being in any

[95]

way the dynamic of true social functions, are more or less characteristic vices contingent upon each kind of creative vision.

It is also true that the love of the mother and the memory of the bliss of intra-uterine life have some relation to the love of the community and its culture, in symbols such as mother country, Alma Mater and Mother Church. These conceptions of the spirit, however, have a quality of conscious inspiration and reason which is utterly unlike the return to sexuality. No kind of social usefulness can be traced to the pursuit of death under the sexual symbol. That which gives sanity and the enjoyment of valuable activity can, however, be naturally derived from the striving of the ego towards self-affirmation and supremacy. In the idea of oneself, so far as it is purged of neurotic ambition, the hope of power directly implies something to rule over, the hope of love implies something to serve. The individual is naturally and necessarily wedded to the community, the self to the world, in a union which has its creative hope and possibility of an altogether reasonable kind.

This is the true dynamic of culture and social

life, man's idea of himself among the rest, his spiritual individuality. It cannot be called an emotion, although it is indeed the prevailing passion of the life, however imperfectly it may be coming to expression. It rules the emotions as with a rod of iron. When we see any man in the grip of emotions, or enduring the pain of their prolonged repression, we may be sure that his ecstasy, suffering and patience are all alike means by which the whole of his being is working its way to his idea of self-value, either usefully, to self and to others, or neurotically, to himself alone.

G

CHAPTER VI

PSYCHOLOGY AND THE CONDUCT OF LIFE

ADLER recommends the study of Individual
Psychology not only to doctors, but generally
to laymen and especially to teachers. Culture
in psychology has become a general necessity,
and must be firmly advocated in the teeth
of popular opposition to it, which is founded
upon the notion that modern psychology
requires an unhealthy concentration of the
mind upon cases of disease and misery.
It is true that the literature of psycho-
analysis has revealed the most central
and the most universal evils in modern
society. But it is not now a question of
contemplating our errors, it is necessary
that we should learn by them. We have
been trying to live as though the oul of
man were not a reality, as though we could
build up a civilized life in defiance of psychic

[98]

truths. What Adler proposes is not the universal study of psycho-pathology, but the practical reform of society and culture in accordance with a positive and scientific psychology to which he has contributed the first principles. But this is impossible if we are too much afraid of the truth. The clearer consciousness of right aims in life, which is indispensable to us, cannot be gained without a deeper understanding also of the mistakes in which we are involved. We may not desire to know ugly facts, but the more truly we are aware of life, the more clearly we perceive the real errors which frustrate it, much as the concentration of a light gives definition to the shadows.

A positive psychology, useful for human life, cannot be derived from the psychic phenomena alone, still less from pathological manifestations. It requires also a regulative principle, and Adler has not shrunk from this necessity, by recognizing, as if it were of absolute metaphysical validity, the logic of our communal life in the world.

Recognizing this principle, we must proceed to estimate the psychology of the individual in relation to it. The way in which an individual's inner life is related to the communal being is distinguishable in three " life-attitudes ", as they are called —his general reactions to society, to work and to love.

By their feeling towards society as a whole —to any other and to all others—man and woman may know how much social courage they possess. The feeling of inferiority is always manifested in a sense of fear or uncertainty in the presence of society, whether its outward expression is one of timidity or defiance, reserve or over-anxiety. All feelings of innate suspicion or hostility, of an undefined caution and desire for some concealment, when such feelings affect the individual in social relations generally, evince the same tendency to withdraw from reality, which inhibits self-affirmation. The ideal, or rather normal, attitude to society is an unstrained and unconsidered assumption of human equality unchanged by any in-equalities of position. Social courage de-pends upon this feeling of secure member-ship of the human family, a feeling which depends upon the harmony of one's own life. By the tone of his feeling towards his neighbours, his township and nation and to other nationalities, and even by his reactions when he reads of all these things in his newspaper, a man may infer how securely his own soul is grounded in itself.

The attitude towards work is closely dependent upon this self-security in society. In the occupation by which a man earns his share in social goods and privileges, he has to face the logic of social needs. If he has too great a sense of weakness or division from society, it will make him unable to believe that his worth will ever be recognized, and he will not even work for recognition : instead, he will play for safety, and work for money or advantage only, suppressing his own valuation of what is the truest service he can render. He will always be afraid to supply or demand the best, for fear it may not pay. Or he may be always seeking for some quiet backwater of the economic life, where he can do something just as he likes himself, without proper consideration of either usefulness or profit. In both cases it is not only society that suffers by not getting the best service : the individual who has not attained his proper social significance is also deeply dissatisfied. The modern world is full of men, both successful and unsuccessful in a worldly sense, who are in open conflict with their occupation. They do not believe in it, and they blame social and economic conditions with some real justice ; but it is also a fact that they have often had too little courage to fight for the best value in their economic function. They were afraid to claim the right to give what they genuinely believed in, or else they felt disdainful of the service society really needed of them. Hence they pursued their gain in an individualistic or even furtive spirit. We must, of course, recognize that so much is wrong in the organization of society, that, besides the possibility of making mistakes of judgment, the individual who is determined to render real social service has often to face heavy opposition. But it is precisely that sense of struggle to give his best which the individual needs no less than society benefits by it. One cannot love a vocation which does not afford some experience of victory over difficulties, and not merely of compromise with them.

It is the third of these life-attitudes—the attitude to love—which determines the course of the erotic life. Where the two previous life-attitudes, to society and to work, have been rightly adjusted, this last comes right by itself. Where it is distorted and wrong it cannot be improved by itself apart from the others. Although we can think how to improve the social relations and the occupation, a concentration of thought upon the individual sex-problem is almost sure to make it worse. For this is far more the sphere of results than of causes. A soul that is defeated in ordinary social life, or thwarted in its occupation, acts in the sex-life as though it were trying to obtain compensation for the kinds of expression of which it fails in their proper spheres. This is actually the best way in which we can understand all sexual vagaries, whether they isolate the individual, degrade the sexual partner or in any way distort the instinct. The friendships of an individual also are integral with the love-life as a whole; not, as the first psycho-analysts imagined, because friendship is a sublimation of sexual attraction, but the other way about. Sexual compulsion—sex as an insubordinate psychic factor—is an abnormal substitute for the vitalizing intimacy of useful friendships, and homosexuality is always the consequence of incapability for love.

The meaning and value which we give to sensations are also united closely with the erotic life, as many good poets have testified. The quality of our feeling for Nature, our response to the beauty of sea and land, and to significances of form and sound and colour, as well as our confidence in scenes of storm and gloom, are all involved with our integrity as lovers. The æsthetic life, with all it means to art and culture, is thus ultimately derived, through individuals, from social courage and intelligent usefulness.

We ought not to regard the communal feeling as something to be created with difficulty. It is as natural and inherent as egoism itself, and indeed as a principle of life it has priority. We have not to create, but only to liberate, it where it is repressed. It is the saving principle of life as we experience it. If anyone thinks that the services of 'busmen, railwaymen and milk-men would be rendered as well as they are without the presence of very much instinctive communal feeling he must be suspected of a highly neurotic scheme of apperception. What inhibits it is, to speak bluntly, the enormous vanity of the human soul, which is, moreover, so subtle that no professional psychologist before Adler had been able to demonstrate it, though a few artists had divined its omnipresence. All unsuspected as it often is, the ambition of many a minor journalist or shop-assistant, to say nothing of the great ones of the world, would be enough to bring about the fall of an arch-angel. Every feeling of inferiority that has embittered his contact with life has fed the imagination of greatness with another god-like assumption until, in many cases, the fantasy has become so inflated as to demand not even supremacy in this world for its appeasement, but the creation of a new world altogether, and to be the god of it. This revelation of the depth of human nature is verified, not so strikingly from the study of cases of practical ambition, however Napoleonic, as from those of passive resistance, procrastination, and malingering, for it is these which show most clearly that an individual who feels painfully unable to dominate the real world will refuse to co-operate with it, at whatever disadvantage to himself, partly in order to tyrannize over a narrower sphere, and partly even from an irrational feeling that the real world, without his divine assistance, will some day crumble and shrink to his own diminished measure.[1]

The question is thus raised, how should we act, knowing this tendency to inordinate vanity in the human soul, and that we dare not merely add to that vanity by assuming ourselves to be miraculous exceptions? Adler's reply is that we should preserve a certain attitude to all our experience, which he calls the attitude of "half-and-half".

---

[1] In case this should seem an exaggeration, we may recall the fact that nearly all the narrowest kind of sects, religious or secular, have a belief in world-catastrophe: the world from which they have withdrawn, and which they despair of converting, is to be brought to destruction, and only a remnant will survive, who will be of their own persuasion.

Our conception of normal behaviour should be to allow the world or society, or the person with whom we are confronted, to be somehow in the right equally with ourselves. We should not depreciate either ourselves or our environment ; but, assuming that each is one-half in the right, affirm the reality of ourselves and others equally. This applies not only to contacts with other souls, but to our mental reactions towards rainy weather, holidays or comforts that we cannot afford, and even to the omnibus we have just missed.

Rightly understood, this is not an ideal of difficult and distasteful humility. It is in reality a tremendous assumption of worth, to claim exactly equal reality and omnipotence with the whole of the rest of creation, in whatever particular manifestation we may be meeting with it. To claim less than this is a false humility, for what results from any contact we make does in fact depend for half its reality upon the way in which we make it. The individual should affirm his part in everything which occurs to him, as his own half of it.

This is often a particularly difficult counsel

to keep in relation to the occupation. In their business, people face more naked realities than are usually allowed to appear in social life ; and it is often almost impossible to allow equal validity to one's own aims and to the conditions of a disorganized world. To do so, means the admission that conditions, just such as they are, are one's real problem—and, indeed, one's proper sphere of action. The division of labour, logical and useful as it is in itself, has given opportunity for human megalomania to create entirely false inequalities, distinctions and injustices, so that we live in an economic disorder which will hardly hold together. To such crazy conditions, the best of men often find it difficult to oppose themselves with perseverance, equally granting its reality and working for its reform. They are tempted to acquiesce in disorder by some inner subterfuge, or to devote themselves to superficial remedies which evade the real problem ; and sometimes they treat their work-life as an unavoidable contamination by things inherently squalid, quite unaware that such an attitude makes them conceited, haughty and, in a profound sense, unscrupulous. It occurs to very few that the right way would be to make alliance on human grounds with others in the same predicament and profession, to assert its proper dignity as a social service and improve it ; but this is the only way in which the individual can really be reconciled with his economic function. Many of those who complain most about the conditions prevailing in their work are doing nothing whatever to reorganize it as a function of human life, and never think of attacking the anarchic individualism which is its ruin. We derive it from Individual Psychology, as a categorical imperative, that every man's duty is to work to make his profession, whatever it may be, into a brotherhood, a friendship, a social unity with a powerful morale of co-operation, and that if a man does not want to do this his own psychological state is precarious. It is true that now, in many professions, the task that this presents is terribly difficult. It is all the more essential that the effort should be made towards integration. For a man's work will never liberate the forces of his psyche unless he is striving, in a large sense, to make it the expression of his whole being, and his idea of his profession must be not only an executive in which he has independence of action, but also a legislative in which he has some authority of direction. In a man's business life the half-and-half valuation leads equally to recognition of reality and to struggle with it by the only realistic method, which is necessarily co-operative.

The pedagogic principles of Individual Psychology, infallible as far as they go, are useless without this practical work of social organization. What has been written above of an individual's duty in his occupation applies in a large sense to his entire social function. A person's function includes active membership of his nation and of humanity, to say nothing of his family. There is a certain parliament which rises for no vacation, and to whose decisions all elected assemblies must in the end defer. It meets in schools, markets, and everywhere on sea and land, for it is the Parliament of Man, in which every word or look exchanged, whether of courtesy or recrimination, of wisdom or folly, has its measure of importance in the affairs of the race. It is everyone's interest to make this wide assembly more united and its discussion more intelligible, for none of us has any real human existence except by reflection from it. When its conclaves are peaceful, all our lives are heightened in tone, health and wealth accrues and arts and education flourish ; when its conversation is reserved and suspicious, work fails, men starve and children languish. In the heat of its dissensions we perish by the million. All its decrees, by which we live or die, and grow or decay, are rooted in our individual attitudes towards man, woman and child in every relation of life.

When we face, objectively, this fact of the relation of all souls and their mutual responsibility, what are we to think of the inner confusion of the neurotic? Is it not simply a narrowing of the sphere of interest, an over-concentration upon certain personal or subjective gains? The neurotic soul is the result of treating the rest of humanity as though its life and aims were altogether of less importance than one's own, and thus losing interest in any larger life. Paradoxically, it often happens that a neurotic has very large schemes of saving himself and others. He is intelligent enough to try to compensate his real sense of isolation and impotence in the human assembly, by a fantasy of exaggerated importance and beneficent activity. He may want to reform education, to abolish war, to establish universal brotherhood or create a new culture, and even plans or joins societies with these aims. He is defeated in such aims, of course, by the unreality of his contact with others and with life as a whole. It is as though he had taken a standpoint outside of life altogether and were trying to direct it by some unexplained magic.

Modern city life especially, with its intellectualism, gives unlimited scope for the neurotic thus to compensate his real unsociability with imaginary messianism, and the result is the disintegration of a people full of saviours who are not on speaking terms.

What is needed, of course, is something very different. It is not that the individual should renounce messianism; for it is a fact that a share of responsibility for the whole future of the race is his alone. It is only necessary that he should take a reasonable view of his power to save society, correctly viewed from his own standpoint : he must become able to regard his immediate personal relations and his occupation as if *they* were of world-importance, for in fact they are so, being the only world-meaning an individual has. When they are chaotic or wrong, it is because we do not, in day-to-day experience, treat them as things of universal meaning. We sometimes treat them as important, no doubt, but generally in a personal sense only.

This tendency of the modern soul, to narrow the sphere of interest, both practically and ideally, is most difficult to subdue, because it is reinforced by the scheme of apperception. For that reason an individual alone cannot do it, excepting only in rare cases. He needs conference with other minds, and an entirely new kind of conference. A resolution to treat one's immediate surroundings and daily activities as if they were the supreme significance of life brings an individual immediately into conflict with internal resistances of his own, and often with external difficulties also, which he cannot at once understand and which no others could rightly estimate unless they were making the same experiment. Hence, the practice of Individual Psychology demands that its students should submit themselves to mutual scrutiny, each one to be estimated by the others as a whole personality. This practice, striking at the root of the false individualism which is the basis of all neurosis, is naturally very difficult to initiate. Upon its success, however, depends the whole future of psycho-analysis as an influence in life at large, outside of clinics and consulting rooms.

In Vienna the work of such groups has already made itself felt in education. The co-operation it has established between teachers and medical practitioners has revolutionized the work of certain schools, and established an equality between teachers and pupils and between pupils themselves, which has cured many children of criminal tendencies, dullness and laziness. Abolition of competition and the cultivation of encouragement have been found to liberate

the energy of both pupils and teachers.
These changes are already affecting the
surrounding family life, which comes into
question immediately the child is psychologically considered. Education, though
naturally the first, is not the only sphere
of life which ought to be invaded by the
activity of such groups. Business and
political circles, which experience the dead-
lock of modern life most acutely, need to
be vitalized with knowledge of human
nature, which they have forgotten how to
recognize.

It is for this work of releasing a new
energy for daily life and its reformation,
that Alfred Adler has founded the International Society for Individual Psychology.
The culture of human behaviour which
this work has begun already to propagate
might well be mistaken for an almost plati-
tudinous ethics, but for two things—its
practical results, and the background of
scientific method out of which it is appear-
ing. In his realistic grasp of the social
nature of the individual's problem and his
inexorable demonstration of the unity of
health and harmonious behaviour, Adler

resembles no one so much as the great Chinese thinkers. If Europe is not too far gone to make use of his service, he may well come to be known as the Confucius of the West.